IT'S TIME FOR YOU TO SHINE

Dear Adisyn,

You are stronger than you know!

Keep shining!

It's Time for You to Shine

A Story of Finding Strength in the Midst of Anxiety and Fear

JENNIFER S. THOMAS

Chameleon O'Clock

It's Time for You to Shine
Finding Strength in the Midst of Anxiety and Fear

Copyright © 2023 by Jennifer S. Thomas

www.chameleonoclock.com

ISBN/SKU 979-8-218-25984-6
EISBN 979-8-218-25985-3

First Printing, 2023

Cover Photo by Shanna Paxton Photography

I dedicate this book to my husband, Leo, and my children, Richard, Samantha, Ethan, Iris, and Christian. Even through my anxiety and fears in life, you always stood by me. Thank you for loving me, even through the darkest of times. I love you.

Mom, I love you. Thank you for being the strong, independent and selfless woman you are!

Lily Pads
Cassandra
Abigail

Contents

Foreword

In the quiet corners of our minds, beneath the tapestry of our experiences, lie the profound stories that define who we are. The journey of self-discovery is a treacherous but transformative one, where the shadows of our anxieties often obscure the light of our true selves. The pages you are about to embark upon chronicle such a journey – a pilgrimage through the labyrinth of anxiety and emergence into self-acceptance.

Anxiety can be overwhelming, like an anchor threatening to drag us into the depths. Yet, as you'll discover in these pages, it can also be a catalyst for remarkable growth. It challenges our limits, questions our beliefs, and forces us to confront the uncomfortable truths that lie within. It is within these uncomfortable truths that we uncover our authentic selves.

As you delve into the author's candid and raw account, you'll share in her experience of navigating anxiety across her life's milestones. The ups and downs, the doubts and breakthroughs – all contribute to a mosaic that captures the essence of human vulnerability and strength. It's a reminder that in our struggles, we are not alone.

But this is not a tale of despair. It's a story of resilience, of one person's unwavering commitment to excavating their potential from the depths of uncertainty. Through introspection, perseverance, and the support of family, they find their way to the surface, breathing in the pure air of self-acceptance and renewal.

Dear reader, may these words serve as both a compass and a mirror. Amidst the constant bombardment of gilded social media lives, may this book guide you through your own uncharted territories and remind you that, even in the midst of life's tumultuous storms, there is a beacon of hope within. The journey towards self-discovery is not without its challenges, but it is a journey worth taking.

And to my dear friend and colleague, Jen, bravo. You are brave. You are kind. And you belong.

Jennifer Sonney, PhD, APRN, PPCNP-BC, FAANP, FAAN

Introduction:
Who AM I?

Who am I? What a loaded question, am I right? Honestly, on any given day my answer to this question used to vary, and I am pretty certain it has for you too. For a long time I thought I knew who I was. I was the mom to my beautiful children, an active duty military spouse to my amazing (and dashingly handsome) husband, a nurse, a researcher, a servant leader, and an advocate. While all of these were definitely parts of my identity and parts I was extremely proud of, they were just small pieces that helped form the big picture of who I truly was.

In all honesty, I only just recently realized who I was, which makes me chuckle because I have studied and published studies on identity in the past. I have taken some really deep dives into understanding what identity crisis is, and you would think that with what I have learned, studied, and published I could clearly answer the question of exactly who I was without hesitation. But I couldn't, not until this one life-changing experience. On a particular day in June of 2023, I became my own hero. I did something that allowed me to conquer my fears and metaphorically kick anxiety in the ass. I felt something in me that I never felt before. Something sparked deep in the core of my being. Something I am still not quite able to explain even now, but I will try my hardest to throughout this book.

I hope that the journey you are about to encounter through my story influences your own unique experience to uncovering your own understanding of who you are. Life is not always beautiful. Life is not always happy. But life is a journey and how you embark on that journey will reveal just how deep you are willing to go in order learn who you really are.

Chapter One

The Decision to Jump

It took me over three years to say yes. The constant cycle of what ifs caused me to hit the brakes every single time. The fear and the anxiety of what could happen, and the sheer lack of control I would have without any safety net in place took over my every waking thought and every cell in my body was in full rebellion. There was absolutely no way I would ever do anything like this... ever.

On May 25, 2023, I was asked the question again. Tori and I crossed paths at countless military functions over the past three years and at each one she asked if I would like to go skydiving. My responses ranged from, "Never!" to "There is no way in hell you could get me to do that!" Each time there was some politeness to my "no," but as I got to know Tori, I became more and more frank with my responses... until May 25, 2023.

We had just finished celebrating my husband's promotion to Lieutenant Colonel, followed by a pretty emotional retirement ceremony. He dedicated 24 years of his life to the military; I spent 23 of them right by his side. So while both the promotion and subsequent retirement were extremely meaningful, the retirement aspect hit a bit deep for all of us. During our time mingling, I saw Tori walking my way. We greeted each other as we always did with her saying, "Hi. How are you? How are the kiddos? Are you ready to jump?" But, this greeting felt different... to me at least. It is hard for me to share this feeling with you without sharing a little glimpse into my backstory. Now, it might seem strange, but I am actually going to take you all the way back to my childhood before describing what this moment felt like and its significance in the plot line of my life.

Childhood

I would like to first preface this childhood reflection with the fact that I had amazing parents! I remember so many fond memories like going to the marina, going crabbing and fishing, camping in the Poconos every

4th of July, and massive family get-togethers during holidays. My dad was born and raised in northern New Jersey and my mom immigrated to the US from the Philippines when she was 22 years old. She and my father had this unbelievable love story of meeting through military friends, becoming penpals, falling in love, and then eventually getting married.

I grew up in Central New Jersey, not too far from Fort Monmouth. That was my father's last duty station and he medically retired from the installation when I was around 3 or 4 years old. To continue to be able to access military services after his retirement, my parents decided to settle around that area. I grew up in the same house for as long as I can remember. I went to the same school district from Kindergarten on. I didn't experience major upheavals in my childhood. Each year followed the same routine from the last. I knew exactly which school I would go to, where the bus would pick me up, and a general idea of the peers I could expect to see in my classes.

I am still amazed at how long I could be around the same groups of people in school and yet I never truly felt a sense of belonging. I never really felt like I fit in. I remember having a few different groups of friends, but till this day (I am 42), I can honestly say I do not have even one friend I keep in touch with regularly at all from my school years. I do get to connect with many on social media, but aside from the occasional greetings I do not have regular contact with anyone. I do not have a childhood best friend.

I remember having a playful childhood, spending hours and hours outside with some of the neighborhood kids. Kickball and SPUD got pretty intense on some of the summer nights. Playing hide-and-seek in the dark was always a family favorite. My dad LOVED to scare us. My sisters and I used to go on bike rides around the neighborhood. I had this light blue bike with a banana seat, and blue and white sparkly streamers hanging from the handlebars. All these fond memories are ones that I keep right at the surface. In a large pond, these memories would be all the lily pads floating serenely at the very top of the pond. These are so easy to access and to remember. But like every pond, there is water underneath those pads. Water that may be murky and that may hold things that cannot be easily seen when just gazing at the surface.

I don't really like to dig or find things at the bottom of bodies of water, no matter how big or small. Something about the dark and just not being able to see through unfamiliar water is not very appealing to me. I find the same theory applies to not so happy memories too. Not delving too much into the details, there were things that I experienced during my childhood that caused me so much pain that I buried the shit out of it. In fact, I not only buried the memories,

I actually took the memories, wrapped them in a garbage bag, placed them into a safe, threw away the key, then threw it into a really deep pond (all metaphorically speaking). Soon after, the lily pads covered the top of it. That was my safety! Having a blanket of amazing memories at the top was definitely my way of staying in control. I believed that as long as the bad memories lurked out of sight at the bottom of the pond, then I could make myself believe that I did not actually experience them. I felt like I had so much control making the choice to bury them so deep and did a really great job at making sure those memories were stuck in time that I actually "forgot" about them. I mean, you don't ever *really* forget a traumatic experience, but somehow you do... until something or someone makes it surface.

The desire to hide this memory from myself and to protect myself from others around me was actually the first and earliest point in my life I can remember experiencing major symptoms of anxiety. Of course, I wasn't aware that's what it was at the time, but as an adult I realized just how intense those symptoms were. The years to follow only amplified those feelings. I had no control over what I experienced, but I was able to control where I put those memories... weighted down at the very bottom of the pond.

Adolescence

If there was one period in my life I wish I could just erase all together it would have to be my adolescence. I was a good kid, but I found myself a little lost for a brief moment in time. During my freshman and sophomore years in high school I did what I could to keep my grades up, but I also did some stupid shit. Again, I was a good kid, but even good kids slip up and make dumb decisions sometimes.... like throwing a massive party at a friend's house while her parents were out of town or staying out three hours past curfew. Those were the two biggest oopsies I did in those early years that I really regret, but I also know that they were great learning experiences. Of course the learning part did not happen until I was an adult and past that obnoxious, know-it-all stage; but I realize that now and I am grateful for the forgiveness and the second chances I received.

During the latter half of my sophomore year I made the decision to enroll in a vocational nursing program. This allowed juniors and seniors to attend nursing assistant and pre-nursing classes, while still in high school. Nowadays, this education method is pretty popular, but it was very new two and a half decades ago. My parents were excited and so proud of me, especially my father.

The summer before entering my junior year, my father became very ill. He spent nearly 60 days in the ICU. I still remember the walk to the elevators at Monmouth Medical Center. Those who worked in the cafeteria already knew us by name by the middle of that summer. I visited my dad a lot, but often felt scared going into his room. I wasn't scared of my father, I was scared about what I did not know. I didn't know just how sick he was and I didn't know that he would never make it back home. He was admitted to the hospital in June and on August 10th my sisters, brother and I were all called to stay at the hospital. My father had taken a turn for the worse. Before being wheeled off to surgery, I remember all of us being rushed into his room just to tell him we love him. As I walked around the side of his bed, I saw the blood pooling on the floor. Now that I am a nurse, I realize he was experiencing disseminated intravascular coagulation (DIC) from sepsis. But as a 16-year-old girl, all I saw was the man I loved so much dying in front of me.

We spent the night in the waiting area, falling asleep pretty late. I remember us being woken up early by my mom. She started by sharing how brave Daddy was during surgery and that he made it out. She then took a pause and I can clearly remember her stating, "and now God is taking care of him." I didn't put two and two together at that moment. My older sister screamed. The others yelled. I just remember looking out the window at how beautiful the sunrise was. I heard the crying, I heard the noise, but I didn't feel anything. Not a tear came from my eye. A moment later, my mom sat right in front of me, blocking my gaze out the window. She started to say, "Jen, are you ...." but before she could finish her question, I took this huge gasp of air. It was like I was holding my breath and did not even know it. I threw my arms around her and began wailing. Everything that immediately followed was an absolute blur.

Shortly after processing that our father had died, we were allowed to see him one last time before we left the hospital. I remember walking in the room and coming alongside his bed. His eyes were closed, but still slightly opened enough to see that his eyes were hazel that morning. His body felt a little cold to me. I remember whispering in his ear that I loved him and if he could please wake up. He didn't. I never mentioned any of these memories out loud... ever. I have come to realize that I buried them at the bottom of the pond. I cannot describe why I did that just yet, but I will say that his passing was single-handedly the greatest devastation I ever experienced in my life.

Over the next couple years, I struggled immensely. I heard many things after my father passed that were devastating to hear and still incredibly hard for me to let go of. As a 16-year-old girl, I was pretty naïve and when someone I loved and trusted told me that my father probably got sick because my siblings and

I were not great kids, I believed them. I can remember the exact location, the exact age I was, and the facial expression of the person saying it to me. In that moment and for many years to follow, I believed that I had control over my behavior and that it was not good enough to keep my father alive.

It was around this time that I began yearning for more acceptance and love, no matter where it came from. The powerful impact my 16th year of life had on me is pretty unbearable to think about still. My father passed away. I felt like I was part of the reason he was sick. The sheer amount of anxiety I was experiencing was overwhelming. But someone noticed me. Someone who was "popular" and well known. And suddenly, I felt loved (or at least that's what I thought at the time). I also felt like I fit in a little more because I was dating this person. But all of that did not last too long. The feelings that is, not the relationship. The relationship actually lasted for a couple years and those couple of years were some of the hardest I ever experienced in my lifetime.

Like many other events that I experienced in my childhood, this is quite hard to think back on. I get choked up remembering what I went through, especially now that I have teenage girls. This is definitely a bottom of the pond memory. I was in so much pain from the abuse and trauma I experienced in that relationship. During that time I had no control over anything. I was controlled by someone else. I could not go anywhere, see anyone, or do anything without getting permission. If I was even a minute late, I was interrogated. There were many times I feared for my life, but felt trapped, scared, and completely lost. Somehow, by the grace of God, I was able to walk out of that relationship after two and a half years of abuse.

While the lack of control and abuse I experienced in that relationship was bad, my pursuit for safety after leaving added to the level of mistrust I had in adults that I thought were supposed to protect me. I filed for a restraining order and was required to appear in court. We (me and my mom's friend) were in a room full of people waiting for their case to be heard and I clearly remember the moment my ex walked through the courtroom door. I lost it. I began hyperventilating and crying hysterically. Just the sheer thought of being in the same room as him scared me to death. The court clerk was able to talk to the judge to see my case first. I sat there in front of the judge and told him what I went through. I begged for a restraining order. I mean, I knew that a protection order wouldn't put up this impenetrable barrier around me, but if I had that in place I could call on the police to keep me safe if the order was ever broken.

After sharing the experiences I went through for what felt like hours, but was really around ten minutes, the judge looked straight at me and asked if I had any proof of the abuse. In that moment a flood of emotions just took over my whole being. I remember having this feeling one time before in my childhood. My word was not enough. The details of the experiences I had were not enough. Me being brave enough to step forward was not enough. He denied my request because I did not have sufficient evidence of abuse. Once again, someone I thought was supposed to protect me didn't believe me. I had no control over this. None. I was devastated.

The man who hurt me tried to contact me a few times after that, even showing up at my house once but I was not home. He did not hurt me again, but it took years, a lot of years, to feel a sense of safety and security around others. I actually still struggle with that quite a bit, but in different ways. I feel this time in my life amplified the anxiety I felt from not having control over what happened to me. Not having control over losing my father. Just not having control over my life period. As I reflect back on this time of my life, I can honestly say that I have a deep-rooted sense of resilience that I didn't know I possessed. If it wasn't for being resilient, I am not sure I would have made it out of those dark years. But iron-clad spine or not, those memories were ones that remained buried at the very bottom of the pond, safe from ever resurfacing... or so I thought.

Early Adulthood and the Years to Follow

I was just 19 years old when I met Leo. My father had passed away some years earlier, but we still had healthcare benefits through the military. Leo, a private in the Army, was a pharmacy tech at the clinic on Fort Monmouth. He had just been assigned there a few months before our paths crossed. How we met and fell in love was not as beautiful as my parents love story, but it did involve Pepto Bismol. My kids love hearing the story and often partake in some kind of reenactment. After meeting Leo, I was determined to get back to the pharmacy so I asked a gastroenterologist I was working for to write a prescription for something for an upset stomach. In the military, everything needed a prescription, even Pepto Bismol. And the rest is history. Our first date was the following night and we have been together ever since.

Leo is a really special guy. He reminded me of my father, someone who perseveres even in the face of adversity. He didn't live the same sort of childhood I did. He grew up in a province in the Philippines, moving to the US when he was 15 years old. He joined the military as a path to college... a path we would soon go on together. Through the first year of our relationship, Leo learned about West Point. By that time he already served a few years as an enlisted soldier. He applied to the Academy, but his acceptance was not smooth sailing. At one point he was told he was not good enough, but through perseverance he showed everyone he was.

One year after beginning a relationship with a man I was madly in love with and who showed me that I am worthy of being treated well, I was dropping him off to the United States Military Academy Prep School. I remember the exact day I did this, as well as every moment of my drive home. I even remember the exact turn I made when I thought to myself that this is just day one of five years being apart. I had no clue if we would make it.

The next five years certainly tested our bond. While Leo was at the Prep School, I graduated with my Licensed Vocational Nursing diploma. When he got to West Point I traveled every weekend I could to see him. It was about a two-hour drive from my house and if I had the opportunity to just see him for 10 short minutes I drove. Cell phones were just becoming popular, while MySpace and AOL Instant Messenger were where everyone was communicating. I could still clearly hear the sound of dial up connections. Ah... the soundtrack of our lives.

We had our fair share of ups and downs through these five years. Perhaps, one of the most trying times of our life and our relationship was when I became pregnant. Leo was just in the second semester of his first year at West Point. We had no clue how we were going to make this work. He was adamant about leaving the Academy to take care of us, but I knew I needed him to stay the course we had decided upon. He worked so hard to be there and while it was going to be hard, I just had this feeling it would all work out in the long run. Richard Anthony Thomas was born in December of Leo's Yuk (sophomore) year. I gave birth one week before graduating with my associate degree in nursing.

Over the next two and a half years Richard and I lived with my mom. A time I could not be more grateful for. She cared for Richard while I worked full time. Till this day, I swear they are soulmates. In turn, I helped to pay bills and did whatever I could to help my mom financially. There was a lot of traveling back and forth for me and Leo to maintain our relationship and so he could build a relationship with Richard even though he was away at school. It was hard, but it paid off. In May 2006, Leo graduated. In June we got married and made our first move across the country. Just like that we took the next big step of our Army life together.

Over the next 17 years, our family grew from three to seven. We moved seven times and lived in 10 different houses. There were so many wonderful experiences we had as a military family. We lived in some amazing areas of the country and met some amazing friends along the way. We visited many places and experienced many adventures. And, we also experienced a lot of hardships.

Leo left on back-to-back-to-back deployments. The first two were in Iraq, the third was in Afghanistan. While being in the Army was a choice and a journey we chose to embark on, it was not easy. Raising my children on my own while my spouse was fighting a war left me feeling lonely and scared that I was going to fail miserably. Moving so much and constantly starting over with my friendships and my career, among many other things, felt like insurmountable tasks each time I experienced it. So, I relied on certain coping mechanisms I developed over the years including: cleaning constantly; organizing and planning everything down to the most minute detail; and doing things that showed I was capable of progressing and achieving great things (i.e.: graduating with my BSN, MSN, and PhD). I did all of this because it allowed me to feel a sense of control over my own environment and they were tangible ways I could show everyone else that I was in control. But was I? As I look back upon that time, I realize that I allowed fear and anxiety to drive my coping mechanism, instead of learning how to cope with living with fear and anxiety.

Present Day

Last year was really rough. I was so consumed by

fear and anxiety that I fell into a deep depression. A couple of things happened that weighed heavily on my heart. Our oldest son was headed to college and I did not feel prepared to let go. But, I did and though it took some time and a small toll on my mental well-being, it was not the event that led me to the state of depression.

With my children getting older, I felt it was a great time to re-enter the workforce as a full-time professional. I worked so hard on my education and I was ready to put it to use. The first year felt awesome and I felt a sense of control over my career that I had never felt before. I got pure joy over the work I was doing and loved the connections I made with those I was serving. Unfortunately, the blissful "honeymoon" phase did not last long as I became a target of bullying and extreme passive aggressive behaviors that impacted the way others perceived me. It was horrible and painful. I suffered from panic attacks and pure shame. I realized just how bad it was when I took part in an assessment that required a diverse group of individuals in and out of the workplace to rate me and a consistent outlier stood out amongst the data (hint: it was the aggressor, who just so happened was also my boss).

I left that toxic environment. I took some time off to try to put it all behind me. Like many other traumatic experiences I faced, I tried to wrap it up, lock it away, and throw it in the bottom of the pond like I had with so many others. I tried many things in an attempt to try and decompress from the strain and stress. Unfortunately, those behaviors I experienced, as well as follow-up behaviors that reared their ugly head did something to my pond. This experience began to stir up some things in the deep dark waters. What I realized was that no matter how meticulously I packed up and tossed the memories and experiences away, they weren't really contained. They just waited at the bottom of the pond for the perfect opportunity to resurface... and they did. They were ugly and painful, and they were contaminating the lily pads. What was once a beautiful surface, was now a murky mess clouded with memories and feelings that I seemingly "forgot" about. This traumatic experience brought back the feelings of trauma, pain, and lack of control I felt in the past, especially with those I trusted, and it began to pull me in.

I swam in that muck, and it was hard to get out. I had a hard time getting out of bed, I gained 25 pounds, I experienced severe mood swings, and at one point I felt I was not good enough or worthy enough for this life. During that time, I allowed fear and anxiety to take over my life in a way I never experienced before. I felt completely out of control for months. But, as I was resilient before, I was resilient again. I found the courage to talk and to seek the help I needed to save me from the pond that was drowning me. This meant intentionally processing those memories I tried so hard to bury and to take control over when and how I would face them. As I processed them one by one, the pond became clearer and I eventually made it out. While there is still some muck left to process, the lily pads bloom along the surface. I am finally able to see the beautiful memories and instead of burying the dark and traumatic memories on the bottom, I have taken control of how they live among the good ones. I took control!

The Decision

So, now that you know a little more about my story, let me take you back to where we first started this book. When Tori and I saw each other at my husband's ceremony, she greeted me as she always did, "Hi. How are you? How are the kiddos? Are you ready to jump?" But, this greeting felt different... to me at least. I didn't have the urge to say no, but I wasn't sure why. A part of me really, really wanted to do this. And then it hit me like a force of a tidal wave. I realized that after months of processing the trauma in my life, I had allowed fear and anxiety to drive my every decision. I processed that new revelation and did not even realize the impact that made in my life, until that very moment. I realized I had control over my decision making process and whether I chose to jump or not, I controlled it... not fear and anxiety. I was in control and I made the fateful decision to jump in with both feet.

Chapter Two

Jump Day

About three weeks had passed since that fateful night and it was jump day. I spent the morning with my girls trying to focus on the why, rather than the nervousness I felt. We went for a jog, and I kept looking up thinking that in a few short hours, I would be free falling from that sky. I am not sure if that helped my nerves or not, but I still got in the car with the family and drove to the hangar. At this point I was still really proud about making the decision to face my fears and jump and knew that this was going to be an iconic experience in my life.

There is an absurd amount of paperwork to sign and initial before you they will allow you to jump out of a plane. All of it was necessary, there was just a lot of it. After completing the paperwork, Tori took me to the dressing area and found a suit that fit well.

The girls and I laughed as most of the suits had holes on the bottom side of them. Lots of butts must have skid along the grass for holes that big to be worn on the suits. As I was suiting up, Tori was giving me the rundown of what to expect. I clearly remember paying very close attention to her every word. Apparently, the serious expression etched on my face showed just how intently I was listening, at least that is what I heard from the kids.

Tori went over processes, elevation, what to expect and many other things. She also shared what I was responsible for, including tucking my head back and bending my knees. To clarify, once we made it to the door of the plane, it was essential that I tucked my head back into Tori's shoulder and bend my knees as if I was trying to touch the bottom of the plane with my heels. Got it. Easy enough. We were going to drive to the runway, get on the plane, takeoff, do our safety checks, scoot to the door, and jump. I was in charge of tucking my head back and bending my knees and Tori would guide the rest.

As the plane began to taxi down the runway, I instantly said to myself, *what the hell am I doing*. I really wanted to shout to stop the plane, but my pride of making it into the plane was the only thing that kept me from making a complete fool of myself before the wheels even left the ground. We started our slow rise up. I remember taking a quick glimpse out the window thinking, *damn that's high.* It was around that time that Tori showed me her wristwatch and said, "We are at about 1,000 feet up." Parts of me felt relieved. Thank goodness. If she is giving me the altitude, then we must be getting ready to get all hooked up. "I will let you know as soon as we get to 8,000 feet so we can start to get hooked up and ready to jump at 15,000." she followed. I know they told me all of this, but the numbers were a total blur as I was looking out the window of this tiny plane. I am pretty sure that if my face was captured in that moment, a meme would have surely been created and would pop up when someone searched "what the f&$# you talking about?"

At 8,000 feet Josh, the cameraman, asked how I was doing. I lied. I said, "A little better," as I looked into the camera. I have watched that video over a hundred times and I can't help but laugh hysterically every single time. I didn't realize just how fake my plastered on smile was. My teeth were clenched together. The corner of my lips did not even point a little upward. Instead, it looked like I just came from the dentist and was shot with Novocain all over. Goodness, I hope that is not what my fake smile really looks like.

We started getting hooked up. I could hear Tori saying all the "checks" out loud behind me. The plane continued to climb higher and higher. *Holy shit, are we there yet??* Was the thought running through my head on a constant loop. If we go any higher I could probably just step right off the plane and onto the moon. A few moments later I began to see the four jumpers sitting ahead of me start to shuffle around. The one nearest to the door was wearing a pair of jeans and sweatshirt, and he had a parachute backpack on. If we were not on a plane I would have thought he was doing something innocuous like going to class. He sat next to the door and made his way onto his knees. He started leaning on the wall of the plane right next to where the door opens and I remember saying to myself, *this idiot. He better back up or he is going to fall out.* Nice one Jen. That is the point.

He began to open the door, holding onto the side looking out. The three other jumpers in front of me were talking and strategizing their positions. And then boom, school boy jumps out and I feel this total numbness take over. In fact, I was secretly hoping I would pass out, but that didn't happen. The three guys in front of me made their way to the door. One was holding the top of the plane while his partners got set. Then I heard, "1...2..." and then silence.

As we inched our way to the wide-open door of the plane 15,000 feet in the air, fear and anxiety took over. What have I done? I can't do this. We needed to scoot up. I could feel my feet making little strides to the door, but they were mainly trying to stop. The problem was that Tori was much stronger than me and even with my little effort, she was able to push me forward incredibly faster than I thought it would go. I kept screaming, "I can't do this. I don't know if I could do this." She kept reminding me I could.

We were poised at the door. I had my chance. Just grab onto the door jamb. They can't force you out! Tori already told me that. So, if I just grab onto the door jamb she would pull me back in. Why weren't my arms moving! Why was I still holding onto the loops of the shoulder strap? Wait.. the jamb. Oh shit, it's happening. Ok, head back and knees bent. I was looking at the Earth from 15,000 feet in the air and all I could think about was head back and knees bent. Then we leapt.

Chapter Three

The Revelation

I suffered with severe anxiety for years and I did not know it until I was well into adulthood. Anxiety, as defined by Oxford, is a feeling of worry, nervousness, or unease, typically about an imminent event or something with an uncertain outcome. Synonyms include worry, concern, and apprehension. According to the Mayo Clinic, signs and symptoms include having a sense of impending danger, panic or doom; gastrointestinal problems, and having the urge to avoid things that trigger anxiety.

Throughout my childhood, I suffered from severe gastrointestinal problems. The military treatment facility we sought care at did every test possible to try and figure out what was physically wrong with me. They tried to figure out what was *physically* wrong with me. By the time I was 12 I had already been hospitalized for observation, had an endoscopy performed, went through a barium swallow and a barium enema, and endured many more invasive exams. I have never had any formal diagnosis as to why my stomach always felt like it was in knots... likely because there was nothing to physically diagnose. I remember these times. I definitely remember the symptoms I was feeling. They were real symptoms, but why were they happening?

After moving through adolescence and into adulthood, I didn't feel those knots nearly as much as I used to. In fact, I forgot that I experienced them at all. Falling in love, growing my family, and working on my education and career definitely allowed me to leave those feelings behind. Not *behind* per se. Just laying at the bottom of the pond.

It wasn't long ago, I built up the courage to ask my mom about those childhood memories. I did not need courage because I thought she would be angry, I needed courage because I did not want to hurt her in any way. She remembers all too well the issues I experienced and even mentioned that some thought I might be a hypochondriac. It wasn't until we really reflected deeply together that we both realized just how much I was unconsciously internalizing the pain I was feeling from the trauma I experienced. I remember going to some counselors, but my mom mentioned I never really opened up to them. I reflect on that a lot and wish I could go back in time and ask those counselors to dig deeper... to not give up on me... to find a way to make me talk. I did not realize just how deep I buried the pain. I mean, I buried it so deep that I even questioned whether some of the experiences even happened.

By now, you are probably wondering how all of this is connected. The trauma, my life experiences, and the skydiving. Well, the skydiving experience was such an life-changing time for me. It was about 7 months before that when I was at my very lowest point in life... feeling I was not worthy to even live. I was in so much pain and I couldn't figure out why. I blamed the trauma I experienced at the job I had left months before that, but in reality it was not solely that experience that made me feel that way. But it was the catalyst that dredged up feelings I felt before in my life and *the* experience that brought me face to face with the unresolved pain lurking at the bottom of the pond. I felt lost, I felt ashamed... and one November night I was thinking deeply about my life and my worth. The thoughts were just raging in my mind like a hurricane. I did the only thing I knew to just get everything I was thinking out. I wrote. I wrote a poem that placed everything I was feeling and all the thoughts going through my head down on paper. I wrote and wrote and wrote until I fell asleep with the journal open next to me and the pen still in my hand.

The next morning I remember waking up with a massive headache and puffy eyes. I cried a lot the night before while I was purging my emotions. Parts of me wanted to visit what I wrote down. Other parts of me was not ready. I am happy I did though, because it wasn't until that morning that I realized just how much I was holding in. I was 41 years old, contemplating life, and only now discovering just how deeply rooted the pain I was feeling was. There were definitely events going on in the present day that were contributing to the day to day anxiety, but it was the bottom of the pond memories that were feeding the anxiety. They were nourishing the anxiety, keeping it alive within me.

Though I do not feel I am ready or will ever be ready to share everything I wrote that night with the world, I am willing to be vulnerable enough to share that there were many self destructive thoughts... thoughts of me not being good enough or worthy enough. But in the midst of that was this little girl wanting to feel heard, an adolescent wishing she had the power to save her father's life, a lost teenager living in so much fear and pain, and a young adult craving control over everything in her life. What I wrote was everything that I was feeling in that moment, valid feelings of unworthiness. But also unresolved feelings of truly traumatic events in my life. But the one piece that kept me going was when I wrote about my children and husband. Not about my role as a mom and a spouse, but about people I live for. They don't know this, but they saved my life.

For the next several weeks I revisited what I wrote often. I just could not believe what I was holding in and when I realized that I could not process this alone, I decided to seek help. I have not had the best of relationships with therapists or mental health providers in the past, but I decided to try again. This time, I put some very intentional effort into finding someone I felt I could connect with. It took a few short weeks of research for me to find that person, and it was worth it. I did not have any amazing revelations after our first visit together. Nor did I have any after our second, third, or fourth. The revelation came when I contemplated and then made the decision to jump with Tori six months later. It was truly surreal and a feeling I will never forget.

Chapter Four

The Experience

The ascent of the plane was pretty much the story of my life. I am excited to do something, I start to do it, I question myself, I fake smile my way through tough feelings, I see others do it, I tell myself I am not good enough, and I resist. And even with all of that, I still placed so much pressure on myself to achieve and over achieve. I accomplished great things and though I am so damn proud of my accomplishments, parts of me know that I did not accomplish those things just for me. I accomplished them because of my desire to prove myself to others. Not anyone in particular, just everyone in general.

I became a very serious person. I had a hard time loosening up throughout my life. Why? Because it allowed me to put up a guard that did not easily let others in, even those I loved most in this world. There were "safe" people I trusted in the past. People who ended up letting me down and because I didn't want to go through that disappointment again, I was sure to be ready and alert. I constantly focused on what I could do next and missed some really important and meaningful times to be present. If each experience was compared to the dive, I would force myself out of the plane not just because I wanted to but mostly because I needed others to know that I could do it.

What I realized that day was that I was not actually afraid of heights... a fear I thought I had for my whole life. Heights were not the problem. What I actually feared was the fall because of the total lack of control I would have, especially over the "what ifs". This is so comparable to life as I was never afraid of getting to where I needed to be. I was afraid of, "What if I fail?" "What if others do not accept me?" "What if I let others down?" What I came to realize was that the anxiety stemmed from what I experienced. It drove each and every one of my actions, the way I behaved. Fear was what I was scared of could happen.

The experiences I had went through during my childhood and adolescence were profound contributors to this fear and the behaviors of control I displayed throughout adulthood. I did a great job covering the pond, so great as a matter of fact that I did not even recognize how the conflicts were impacting me and those around me. As I reflect on my adult life,

I realize that there were times that my pond surface would become tainted and these were the times I felt the least amount of control and exhibited the highest amount of harmful behaviors. Harmful to me and the relationships around me. I see this now. Like they say, hindsight is 20/20. After months of processing I realize just how deeply rooted my behaviors were.

As we made the jump out of the plane I did what any normal person would do. I screamed. Not just any scream. I swear that I exerted every single ounce of energy I had in my lungs towards making this ungodly sound come out of my mouth. In fact, Tori and Josh mentioned they were not sure they have ever had anyone scream for as long as I did. I am not even sure I took a breath. We were moving fast, around 120 miles per hour. The air had a slight chill to it, but that didn't bother me. I could feel the pressure of the air against my face and my skin stretching so far back that I swear the corners of my mouth were nearly touching my ears. It was chaotic, but the sweetest sense of freedom. Approximately one minute later, Tori pulled the cord and the chute deployed. We made a quick rise up and as the chute caught the air we slowly began our decent down.

It took a good minute for me to gather myself. I remember breathing rapidly and some tears dripping from the corner of my eyes. They didn't quite make it down my face as the goggles I was wearing caught them. But as soon as I caught my breath I took it all in. Though I have been on a plane before, I never experienced the beauty of the world like I did in that moment. The rays of the bright sun shined through the white clouds that were in the sky that afternoon. Green hilltops and a snowcapped Mount Rainier was posing in what looked like a backdrop of a movie. But it was all real. I did not forget that I was still up in the air with no safety net. I knew exactly where I was and I was still scared shitless, but I did not let the fear take over the moment as I have done so many times before.

Tori was on jump number 1,100 ish. I was on jump one. She has seen this view hundreds of times, but shared with me that it never gets old. I believe it. The journey towards the ground was full of a few bumps and maybe one time where I screamed, "Please don't drop me!" But the beautiful, serene, cathartic experience represented a major milestone and iconic moment in my life. You see, in life itself there were many times I should have experienced beauty in the moment, but was so wrapped up in the need to control the experience and outcomes that I missed countless opportunities to take it all in. It wasn't until this very experience that I realized that and though I can dwell in the grief of feeling like I was not fully present in the moment, I choose not to. I no longer choose to allow the past to define how I live right now, in the present.

Chapter Five

It's Time for You to Shine

As we continued our decent back towards the Earth, I just continued to take it all in. I wasn't sure I would ever have this experience again, so I breathed in the fresh air, took in the sound of beautiful silence, felt the weightlessness of my body floating in the sky, and just looked at the beautiful sereneness of the Earth rushing around me. As we were approaching the landing area, I put my legs up and Tori leaned back to ensure we had a nice smooth landing. We landed well. I didn't skid much, but I could surely understand why every suit that was available in the dressing area had holes on the bottom side of them.

As we made our way back to the hangar, my husband and kids were outside waiting for me. I had barely started walking towards them when they all surrounded me with hugs, asking me how the experience was. I was still in a state of adrenaline overflow but remember feeling so proud. My kids were so proud. My husband was so proud. I was so proud. I did it.

Till now this book has been totally about me and my experiences. However, it is my hope that through the words you can feel the emotional undercurrent and that they served as an opportunity to connect with yourself in a meaningful way. I write to connect. I write to be real. I write to be human.

While working on my PhD in Nursing, I fell in love with qualitative research and not just any qualitative research. I fell in love with interpretive phenomenology, a value laden approach to understanding people's experiences. I have realized that there is a beautiful connection that can be made between the deep sense of knowing (epistemology) and the deep sense of being (ontology). And through this, there is a sweet connection to identity.

What we experience throughout our lives are tangible moments within reality. How we manage and interpret those tangible moments within reality make detectable and undetectable impacts on our views, our behaviors, our beliefs, our values... our life. But we don't always understand this. We can't understand why some of us have such controlling and overbearing personalities, while others remain timid and prefer to stay in the shadows. But if we can just allow ourselves to truly understand our journeys, we may have an insurmountable impact on the world.

This journey that we call "life" is just that. It is a journey. When we decide on a destination, we take time to think about what we want to experience. How will we get there? What is the price and how long will it take? While we can plan for the most amazing experience, the path to get to where we want to be may change. It might cost some folks more and others less. It may take longer than anticipated, or we may never get there at all. But the focus should not be on the destination. The focus should be on the journey.

Too often we choose the path of least resistance. The path that does not have overbearing weeds of past experiences, hurt, pain, and trauma mixed in with the road that represents love, happiness, and joy. We take the path where we don't have to face those weeds because it is easier, it is faster, it is clearer, and it is safer. But that does not mean that the other path goes away. No, instead the weeds continue to grow and get thicker over time. And at some point, both paths will merge and we will have to begin weeding our way to moving forward. It will be messy. You will get tired. You will want to stop and rest and at times shed a tear. But as you tackle each weed, you will find the path becomes clearer. You will find your way to your destination and will look back at the beautiful path that you cleared while you were finding your way through.

All of this is not meant to say that you will be able to rid yourself of the bottom of the pond memories. Truthfully, they will never go away. But you can take control over how much you will allow those memories to muddy up your pond. You can choose how they live alongside your lily pads. It will take time and effort. Every time you see the pond becoming a little more clear, some sludge from the bottom may rise. But your strength, your perseverance, and your desire to live an amazing life free from the chains of the past will give you the strength needed to keep pushing forward.

So, who are you? That may still be a loaded question, but as you embark on this journey of self-discovery, remember this...

You are beautiful. You are unique.
You are resilient. You are exquisitely you and...

It's time for you to shine!

Reflection and Notes

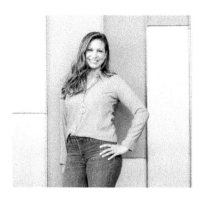

Dr. Jen Thomas is an inspirational storyteller who finds meaningful connections between lived experiences, identity, and behavior. Her personal experiences as a military spouse, mom to biological and adopted children, military mom, nurse, daughter, sister, biracial woman, God-fearing human, trauma survivor, and experiencer of severe burnout has led her to some beautiful life experiences, as well as some very dark times. At her lowest point in life, she found security and comfort in her passion for writing.

Dr. Thomas is a strong and fierce advocate for mental health awareness in both personal and professional settings. She has utilized her experiences, knowledge, and skills to create a coaching, consulting, and motivational speaking firm directed towards helping others build confidence, set and reach goals, and journey towards the best version of themselves.

To learn more about Dr. Thomas' services, visit www.chameleonoclock.com

(Photo Credit: Shanna Paxton Photography)

Printed in the USA
CPSIA information can be obtained
at www.ICGtesting.com
BVHW050944220823
668781BV00002B/15